The Best Mediterranean Cookbook

50 Mouth-Watering Recipes for Your Daily Mediterranean Meals

Jenna Violet

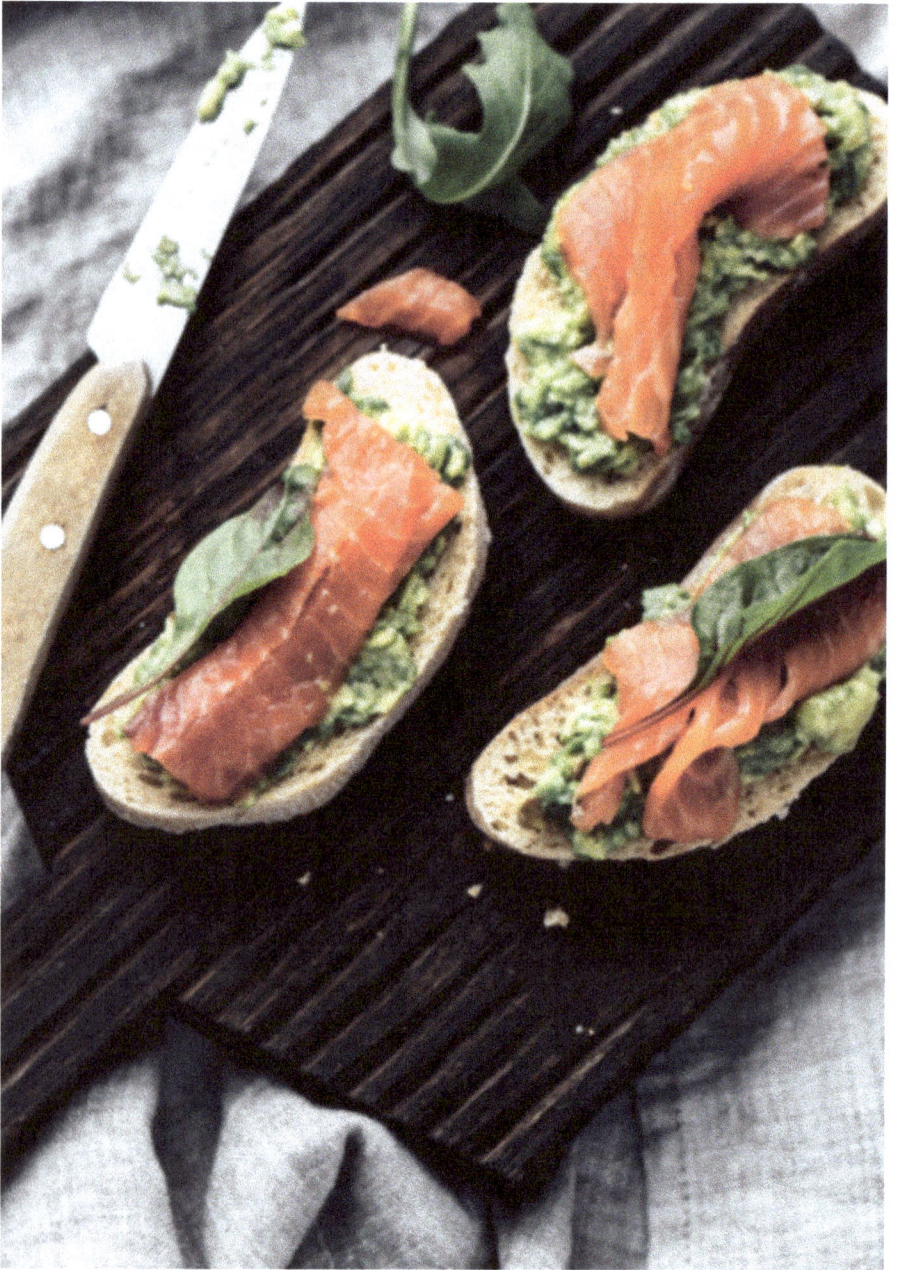

Table of Contents

Wonton soup

Ingredients

- Chopped greens
- 1 leek, white parts, thinly sliced
- Scallions, cilantro, sesame seeds
- 4 slices ginger
- Salt and lemon juice to taste
- 1 tablespoon of olive oil
- 4 cups of chicken broth
- 14 wontons

Directions

- In a medium pot , sauté the shallot with ginger in olive oil, over medium heat, until fragrant.
- Add the broth, cover and bring to a boil.
- Add the wontons and simmer according to directions on the package.
- Taste, and adjust the seasoning accordingly.
- Place in the greens let cook until wilted.
- Spinach and kale take more time compared to others.

- Divide between two bowls, then sprinkle with cilantro, scallions, and sesame seeds.
- Enjoy.

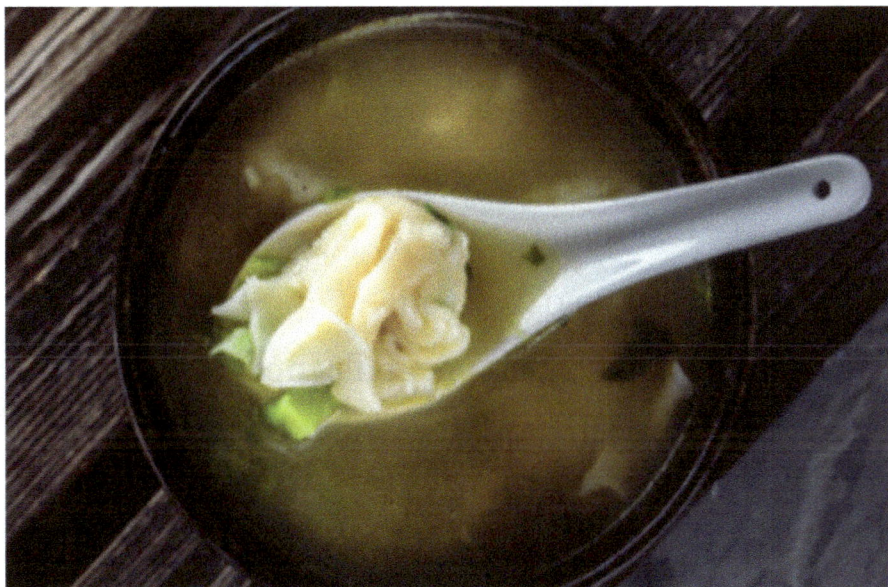

Roasted Portobello steaks with walnut coffee sauce

Ingredients

- 1 teaspoon of miso
- 4 garlic cloves, chopped
- 4 extra-large Portobello mushrooms
- 5 tablespoons of olive oil
- ½ teaspoon of pepper
- ½ teaspoon of salt
- 1 teaspoon of balsamic
- Generous pinch salt and pepper
- 2 extra-large shallots, rough diced
- 1 cup of walnuts, raw
- 1 tablespoon of balsamic vinegar
- 1 ¼ cup of black coffee
- Drizzle of truffle oil , a spring of thyme

Directions

- Preheat oven ready to 400°F.
- Then, mix olive oil together with the vinegar in a small bowl.
- Use it to brush the Portobello on both sides.

- Season, or sprinkle with salt and pepper and place gills side down, on a parchment lined sheet pan .
- Let bake until tender in 25 minutes.
- Wrap in foil until ready to use.
- Heat another olive oil in a medium sauce pan, over medium heat.
- Sauté the shallots with the garlic until fragrant and tender, stirring often.
- Add the walnuts and stir for 2 minutes.
- Add the coffee, scraping up any brown bits.
- Pour into a blender with salt , pepper, miso paste, balsamic.
- Then, blend until silky smooth.
- Place the sauce back in the pan and heat up gently before plating.
- When the Portobello are done, slice and place over the Coffee Walnut sauce in a serving dish .
- Top with a sprig of thyme and pomegranate seeds .
- Serve and enjoy.

Vegan tomato soup with coconut, ginger, and turmeric

Ingredients

- 3/4 teaspoon of salt
- 2 tablespoons of olive oil
- 1 14 ounce can of coconut milk
- 2 fat shallots, rough chopped
- 3 garlic cloves, rough chopped
- Peanut Chili Crunch and Scallions
- 1 tablespoon of ginger, rough chopped
- 1 14 ounces can of diced tomatoes
- 2 teaspoons of fresh turmeric, rough chopped
- 1 cup of water
- ¼ teaspoon of cayenne
- 1 tablespoon of tomato paste

Directions

- Begin by Sautéing the shallot together with the garlic, ginger, and fresh turmeric in a medium pot , over medium heat in olive oil, until deeply golden.
- Add the tomato paste, stir for 1 minute.

- Transfer to a [blender](#) with the can of tomatoes, puree until so smooth.
- Return back to the same pot.
- Add 1 cup of water with can of [coconut milk](#), ground turmeric, [salt](#), and cayenne.
- Bring to a simmer, turn off heat, taste, and adjust the seasoning accordingly.
- Divide among bowls and top with [Peanut Chili Crunch](#) and scallions.
- Serve and enjoy.

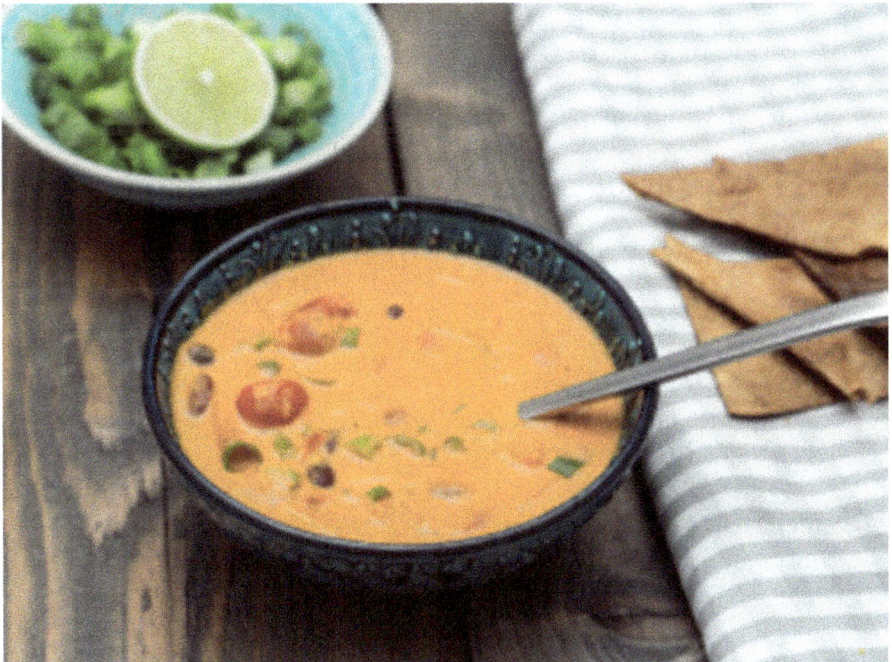

Roasted parsnips with romesco sauce

Ingredients

- 1 teaspoon of cumin
- 3 extra-large parsnips
- ½ teaspoon of chili flakes
- ¾ teaspoon of salt
- 1 red bell pepper, halved
- 1 tablespoon of tomato paste
- ¾ inch thick wedges of onions
- 1 tablespoon of sherry wine vinegar
- Salt and pepper
- 1 teaspoon of smoked paprika
- ¼ cup of chopped fresh Italian parsley
- 2 garlic cloves
- Olive oil
- ¼ cup of water
- ½ cup of toasted hazelnuts

Directions

- Preheat oven to 425°F.
- Place parsnips and bell pepper on a parchment lined sheet pan .

- Add onion wedges to the pan.
- Brush with olive oil all over.
- Season and or sprinkle with salt and pepper.
- Let roast for 35 minutes until fork tender.
- Place bell pepper and onion in a food processor .
- Add remaining romesco ingredients and pulse to form paste.
- The, spoon the romesco sauce onto a platter, smear all over.
- Arrange the parsnips overtop.
- Sprinkle with chopped parsley and crushed hazelnuts .
- Serve and enjoy immediately.

Szechuan chicken and Brussels sprouts

Ingredients

- 1 tablespoon fresh ginger
- 2 lbs. chicken thighs
- 1 teaspoon salt , more for sprinkling
- 1 ½ lbs. medium Brussel sprouts, halved
- 1 tablespoon of sesame oil
- 4 fat garlic cloves, finely minced
- 1 teaspoon of Szechuan peppercorns
- ¼ cup of honey
- ¼ cup of soy sauce
- 1 tablespoon of rice vinegar
- Scallions
- 3 teaspoons of garlic chili paste

Directions

- Preheat oven to 425°F.
- Combine honey, soy sauce, rice vinegar, sesame oil, chili paste, garlic, ginger, salt, and Szechuan peppercorns in a medium bowl.
- Pour *half of the marinade* over the chicken.
- Place and lock in a bag, let marinate.

- Place Brussel sprouts in a bowl, then pour the remaining marinade over Brussel sprouts, toss.
- Nestle the chicken thighs in between, and spoon any remaining marinade over the chicken.
- Season the *chicken with a little salt.*
- *Let b* ake for 30 minutes in the preheated oven, checking at 20 minutes.
- Divide the Brussel sprouts and top with the chicken.
- Sprinkle with scallions.
- Serve and enjoy.

Palak paneer

Ingredients

- ¾ cup of plain yogurt
- 1 paneer
- ½ cup of cashews
- 1 cup of water
- 12 ounces of frozen spinach
- 3 tablespoons of ghee
- Squeeze lemon
- 1 teaspoon of salt
- 1 white onion, diced
- 2 tablespoons of ginger, rough chopped
- ½ teaspoon of sugar
- 4 garlic cloves, rough chopped
- 1 jalapeno
- 2 teaspoons of cumin
- 2 teaspoons of coriander
- 2 teaspoons of Garam masala
- 1 teaspoon of black mustard seeds

Directions

- In a large skillet, heat bit of ghee.

- Season the ghee with salt and pepper.
- Then, pan-sear the paneer until golden and crispy.
- Wipe out the skillet, heat 3 tablespoons of ghee over medium heat.
- Add onion together with the ginger, garlic, and chilies.
- Sauté for 15 minutes, or until deeply golden and fragrant, stirring often.
- Add coriander together with the cumin , Garam masala , and mustard seeds, let sauté 3 more minutes.
- Add the frozen spinach and cup of water, over low heat, simmer uncovered until the spinach is thawed.
- Transfer to a blender , top with the yogurt and cashews.
- Add the salt and sugar , then, blend until silky smooth.
- If salty, add the paneer to soak the salt.
- Place the blended spinach sauce back into the pan uncovered, on med-low heat.

- Add the pan-seared paneer and continue cooking until the paneer is warmed through.
- Serve and enjoy over naan Bread or cauliflower rice .

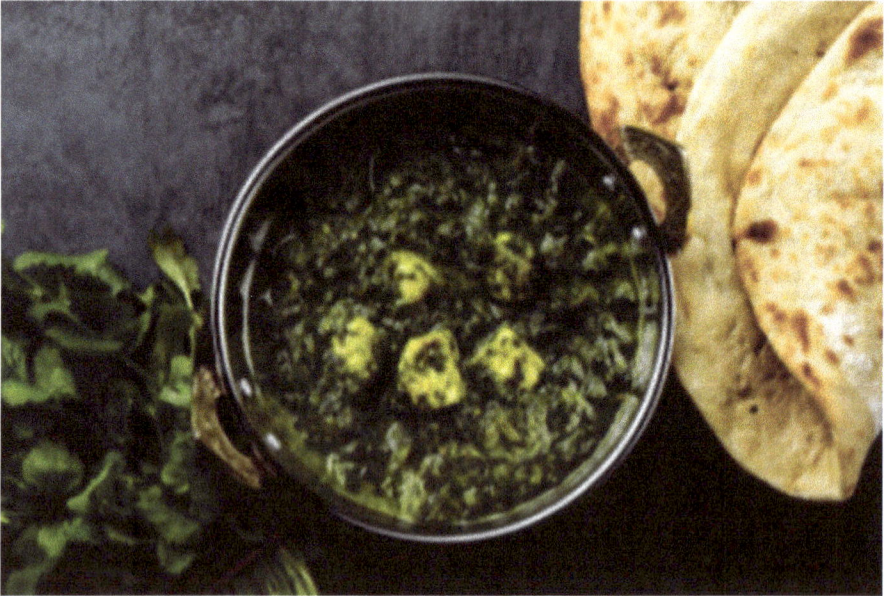

Pressure pot mujadara

Ingredients

- ½ teaspoon of cinnamon
- 1 teaspoon of allspice
- 1 cup of [brown lentils](#)
- lemon zest from 1 small lemon
- 1 ½ tablespoons of olive oil
- 3 cups of water
- 3 fat shallots, thinly sliced
- 4 cloves garlic, rough chopped
- 2 teaspoons of cumin
- ¼ teaspoon of ground ginger
- 1 teaspoons of coriander
- 1 cup of **brown** [basmati rice](#)
- 1 teaspoon of dried mint
- ½ teaspoon of turmeric
- 1 ½ teaspoons of kosher salt

Directions

- Place lentils in a bowl and cover with hot tap water.

- Sauté shallots in olive oil for 5 minutes, stirring constantly.
- *Remove half* , saving for the topping.
- Add the garlic and sauté until fragrant.
- Add all the spices, salt , lemon zest, and water. Stir.
- Drain the lentils and add them with the rice to the pressure pot. Stir.
- Cover, set to h**igh pressure for 11 minutes.**
- Let naturally release for 10 minutes.
- Gently fluff the Mujadara with a fork.
- Divide among bowls, drizzle with olive oil .
- Add tomatoes, avocado together with the caramelized shallots, sprouts, a spoonful of yogurt.
- Enjoy.

Grilled eggplant salad with freekeh and yogurt dressing

Ingredients

- 4 tablespoons of olive oil
- 1 cup of dry freekeh
- 2 ½ cups of water
- Sumac
- 2 garlic cloves finely minced
- ½ teaspoon of pepper
- 1 large eggplant, sliced
- Salt
- 1 cup of plain thick Greek yogurt
- ¼ cup of mint, chopped
- ½ teaspoon of Aleppo chili flakes
- 3 cup of dill, chopped
- ¼ cup Italian parsley, chopped
- 3 scallions, sliced
- 1 tablespoon of lemon zest
- 4 tablespoons of lemon juice

Directions

- Preheat your grill to medium high.

- Then, place freekeh with water in a medium pot.
- Bring to a boil, cover, lower the heat, let simmer for 20 minutes.
- Brush sliced eggplants with olive oil .
- Season with salt, then, grill on both sides for 4 minutes.
- Wrap in a foil, let steam and cook through. Cut into bite-sized pieces.
- Combine cooked freekeh together with the eggplant, lemon zest, scallions, chopped herbs, olive oil , lemon juice, salt , pepper, and spices in a bowl. Toss.
- Taste and adjust the seasoning with salt and lemon.
- Combine yogurt, lemon juice, dill, garlic, sumac, and salt in a small bowl, whisk.
- Serve and enjoy.

Grilled romaine salad with corn, fava beans, and avocado

Ingredients

- 1 tablespoon of lemon juice
- 2 romaine hearts
- 1 ear corn, shucked
- 6 tablespoons of olive oil
- 1 tablespoon of sherry vinegar
- 1 teaspoon of honey
- 1 teaspoon of sumac
- ¼ teaspoon of salt and pepper
- ½ pound fresh fava beans in pods
- 3 tablespoons of chopped dill
- 1 lemon
- ½ pound of shrimp
- 1 avocado, diced
- ½ teaspoon of salt
- 1-pint cherry tomatoes, cut in half.
- ½ cup plain yogurt
- 1 tablespoon lemon juice
- 2 fat clove garlic, finely minced

Directions

- Preheat your grill to medium high.
- Whisk together olive oil, sherry vinegar, lemon juice, honey, sumac, salt, and garlic, set aside.
- Brush the romaine with olive oil.
- Season with salt , then grill each side briefly until grill marks appear on. Keep on a platter.
- Grill the lemon with the corn on the cob, fava beans, and shrimp over medium heat.
- After 10 minutes, shuck and divide among the romaine wedges.
- Cut the kernels off the corn and divide.
- Add the diced avocado and halved cherry tomatoes.
- Squeeze the salad with the grilled lemon halves, spoon a little dressing over top.
- Scatter with fresh herbs.
- Serve and enjoy.

Summer pasta salad with zucchini, corn, and cilantro pesto

Ingredients

- 6 ounces of rice noodles
- ½ teaspoon of smoked paprika
- ½ teaspoon of coriander
- ½ teaspoon salt
- 2 medium zucchini
- ¼ teaspoon of pepper
- 1 red bell pepper
- ½ of an onion
- 2 ears of fresh corn
- 1 tablespoon of lime zest
- ⅓ cup of pumpkin seeds
- Salt and pepper
- 1 large bunch cilantro and thin stems
- 2 fat garlic cloves
- 2 tablespoons of chopped jalapeno
- 2 tablespoons of lime juice
- ½ cup of olive oil

Directions

- Preheat your grill ready to medium high.
- Brush the veggie with olive oil and sprinkle with salt and pepper.
- Pour boiling water over the rice noodles, drain and rinse. Keep aside.
- Place the veggies on the grill, lower heat to medium, cover.
- Place cilantro together with the garlic and jalapeño in a blender, pulse until finely chopped.
- Add the remaining ingredients, pulse to combine. Not so smooth.
- Cut the vegetables into bite-sized pieces, when they are done.
- Loosen the pasta with cold water. Drain in dish.
- Add the Cilantro Pesto with the veggies.
- *Taste, and a* djust the seasoning accordingly.
- Serve and enjoy topped with halved cherry tomatoes and lime wedges.

Lentil salad with spring veggies, mint, and yogurt sauce

Ingredients

- 2 garlic cloves finely minced
- 2 cups of cooked lentils
- 1 lemon, zest and juice
- 3 cups of spring veggies
- ¼ teaspoon of salt
- 2 tablespoons of fresh chopped dill
- Salt and pepper
- ½ teaspoon of sumac
- 3 tablespoons of red onion
- 2 garlic cloves
- ¼ cup of chopped mint leaves
- 2 tablespoons of olive oil
- 1 teaspoon of sumac
- 1 cup of plain thick Greek yogurt
- 1 tablespoon of lemon juice

Directions

- Start by cooking the lentils in salted water until tender.

- Slightly steam the veggies.
- Place the lentils together with the veggies, onion, garlic, and mint in a bowl.
- Toss with the olive oil , lemon zest, and lemon juice.
- Season with salt , pepper, and sumac.
- Mix Greek yogurt, lemon juice, dill, garlic, sumac, and salt in a small bowl
- Smear the yogurt sauce on a platter topping with lentil salad.
- Serve and enjoy.

Creamy polenta with spring veggies and gremolata

Ingredients

- 1 cup of mushrooms
- ½ cup of dry polenta
- 2 cups asparagus
- 1 teaspoon of fresh thyme
- ¾ teaspoon of salt
- 1 teaspoon of granulated onion powder
- ¼ teaspoon of pepper
- 2 ½ cups of water
- 4 tablespoons of olive oil
- 2 tablespoons of gremolata
- 5 cups of veggies
- 1 shallot, chopped
- 1 cup of porcini mushrooms
- 1 cup of fiddlehead ferns
- Handful of pea shoots
- 2 tablespoons of sherry wine
- Salt and pepper

Directions

- Bring water to boil in a medium pot .
- Season with salt , pepper, and spices.
- Gradually whisk in the dry polenta, let simmer for 10 minutes covered over low heat.
- Continue to cook for another 10 minutes.
- Stir in the olive oil. Switch off heat source.
- In a large skillet, heat olive oil over medium heat.
- Add mushrooms, let sauce until tender.
- Add shallot and other veggies.
- Season with salt and pepper, stir.
- Lower heat, continue to cook for 5 minutes until fork tender.
- Serve and enjoy.

Vegan green goddess bowl

Ingredients

- 1 tablespoon of vinegar
- 1 tablespoon of water
- 4 radishes, sliced
- 1 cucumber, sliced into ribbons
- 1 teaspoon of kosher salt
- 10 green beans
- 1 carrot, sliced into ribbons
- 1 tablespoon of lemon
- 3 tablespoons of olive oil
- 1 teaspoon of white miso paste
- 1 avocado, sliced in half
- 1 cup of shelled edamame
- 6 small potatoes
- 10 asparagus spears
- 1 package of *silken* tofu
- 2 fat garlic cloves
- 1 fat scallion, white and green parts
- 1 cup of fresh herbs
- ½ teaspoon of pepper

Directions

- Bring salted water to a simmer on the stove.
- Add the whole potatoes, cover and simmer until fork tender.
- Remove the potatoes, set aside, keep warm.
- Place in the edamame together with the asparagus, and green beans into the same hot water, continue to simmer briefly until tender and bright green. Strain.
- Divide between two bowls and serve with dressing.
- Place silken tofu, garlic, scallion, herbs, olive oil, lemon, vinegar, water, kosher salt, miso, and pepper in a blender.
- Blend until smooth.
- Taste and adjust seasoning.
- Serve and enjoy.

Blackened tempeh with kale and avocado

Ingredients

- 1 scallion, sliced
- ⅓ cup of vegan ranch dressing
- Cajun spice blend
- Pinch salt, lemon zest from ½ a lemon
- ¼ cup of pickled onions
- 1 block tempeh
- 2 tablespoons of olive oil
- 1 avocado, sliced
- 5 leaves of lacinato kale
- 1 teaspoon of oil
- 4 radishes, sliced

Directions

- Firstly, stir the spice into the dressing.
- Taste, and adjust accordingly.
- Add the tempeh, and sauté pan with salted water, enough to cover.
- Let simmer for 10 minutes to reduce bitterness.
- Slice and coat each side with Cajun Spices.

- Then, pan-sear the tempeh in bit of oil, until crispy. Set aside.
- Stack the kale, cut in to thin ribbons.
- Place in a bowl and add a teaspoon, a pinch of salt and lemon zest.
- Massage with your fingers until tender.
- Add the radishes together with the scallion, pickled onion, and avocado to the kale.
- Toss with some of the Vegan Ranch dressing to coat.
- Divide the salad among bowls top with the blackened tempeh and sprouts.
- Serve and enjoy.

Tarragon chicken with asparagus, lemon, and leeks

Ingredients

- 2 large leeks, sliced
- 1 extra-large bunch asparagus
- ½ teaspoon of pepper
- 2 lemons
- 2 teaspoons of salt
- 1/ 4 cup of olive oil
- 6 garlic cloves, finely minced
- 1-ounce package of fresh tarragon leaves
- 1.5 lbs. chicken breast

Directions

- Place the zest of 1 lemon with its juice in a small bowl.
- Then, add olive oil, garlic, salt and pepper, mix until salt dissolves.
- Add ½ of the fresh tarragon, saving the balance for garnish.
- Place the asparagus in a bowl and spoon some of the marinade over top.

- Toss to combine, then place on a parchment lined sheet pan .
- Add leeks to the same bowl, toss with a little marinade and spread out on the sheet pan .
- Add the chicken breasts, with the remaining marinade, coat.
- Nestle the chicken amongst the asparagus.
- Zest the second lemon over the whole sheet-pan, slice the lemons into rounds, layering them over the asparagus.
- Let bake for 20 minutes until golden.
- Remove, toss to coat the chicken top with the flavorful juices.
- Serve and enjoy.

Curry tofu salad

Ingredients

- 3 tablespoons of vegan mayo
- ½ teaspoon of cayenne pepper
- 8 ounces of tofu- extra firm
- 1 tablespoon of olive oil
- ¼ cup of cilantro, chopped
- 1 tablespoon of apple cider vinegar
- ¼ teaspoon of salt and pinch pepper
- ¼ cup of cashews, chopped
- ¼ cup of golden raisins
- ½ cup of celery, chopped
- Salt and pepper
- ¼ cup red onion, diced
- ½ cup of apple, diced
- 1 tablespoon of honey
- 3 teaspoons of curry powder

Directions

- Begin by squeezing any excess water out of the tofu with a paper towel.
- Then, cut into small cubes, blot again.

- In a large skillet heat olive oil over medium heat.
- Add salt and pepper to the olive oil then add tofu.
- Sear on all sides until deeply golden, with a spatula turn, repeatedly.
- Add raisins together with the onions, celery, cashews, apple, cilantro, stir.
- Add spices, vegan mayo honey, and vinegar.
- Season with salt and pepper.
- Stuff into pitas with a handful of greens, or stuff avocados
- Serve and enjoy.

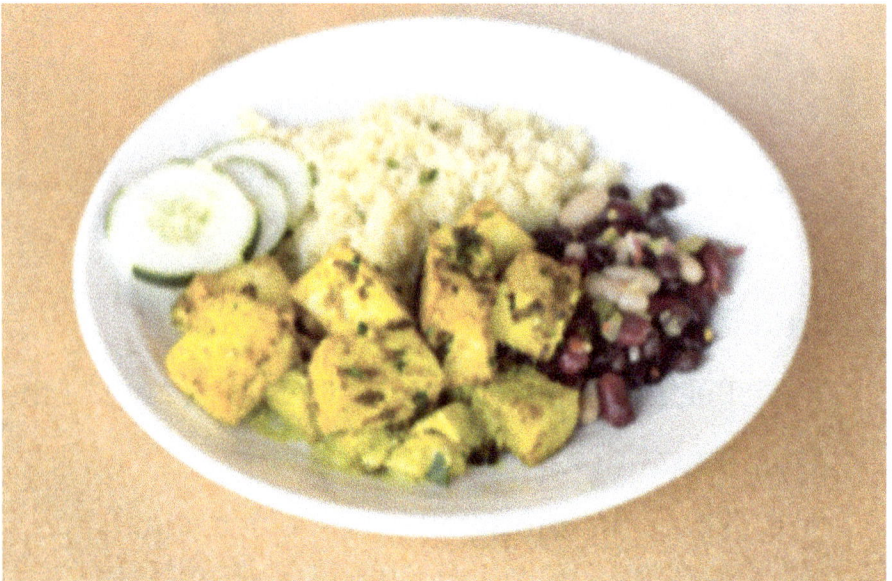

Beet noodles with yogurt and dill

Ingredients

- 1 tablespoon fresh dill, chopped
- 1 tablespoon of olive oil
- Salt and pepper to taste
- 1 fat shallot
- ¼ cup of water
- Toasted pine nuts
- 2 garlic cloves, rough chopped
- 6 ounces of beet noodles
- 3 tablespoons of plain yogurt

Direction

- In a large skillet, heat the oil over medium heat.
- Add the shallot together with the garlic and beet noodles, let sauté for 4 minutes, until golden and fragrant.
- Add the water, let simmer for 6 minutes covered or until beet noodles are tender.
- Uncover and continue to simmer.
- Swirl in the yogurt and stir in the fresh dill.

- Season with salt and pepper.
- Top with toasted pine nuts and fresh dill.
- Serve and enjoy immediately.

Sweet and sour chicken

Ingredients

- Groundnut oil
- 100g of tender stem broccoli
- 1 x 227g tin of pineapple in natural juice
- 100g of baby sweetcorn
- 1 x 213g tin of peaches in natural juice
- 7cm piece of ginger
- ½ a bunch of fresh coriander
- 1 tablespoon of low-salt soy sauce
- 2 teaspoons of corn flour
- 1 yellow pepper
- 2 x 120g of chicken breasts
- Chinese five-spice
- 1 lime
- 2 cloves of garlic
- 1 bunch of asparagus
- 1 small onion
- 2 fresh red chilies
- 1 tablespoon of fish sauce
- 1 red pepper

- 1 teaspoon of runny honey

Directions

- Drain the juices from the tinned fruit into a bowl.
- To it, add the soy and fish sauces, whisk in half of corn flour until smooth.
- Lay chicken skin in a large, cold frying pan, place on a low heat, briefly to render the fat, turning occasionally.
- Remove once golden, add a pinch of sea salt and five-spice.
- Place chunks of the chicken in a bowl together with 1 heaped teaspoon of five-spice, a pinch of salt, 1 teaspoon of corn flour, garlic, and half the lime juice.
- Place a frying pan on a high heat, cook the chicken for 6 minutes, turning halfway, leave on a low heat.
- Place a work on a high heat, scatter in the pepper and onion to scald and char for 5 minutes.

- Add 1 tablespoon of olive oil, ginger, garlic, chilies, peaches, pineapple, baby sweetcorn, asparagus, and broccoli.
- Stir-fry for 3 minutes, pour in the sauce, cook briefly loosening splash of boiling water.
- Drizzle the honey into the chicken pan, raise the heat to high, toss until sticky.
- Serve and enjoy with the coriander leaves and lime wedges for squeezed.

Peanut butter oatmeal cookies

This is a gluten free recipe deliciously worth making at home at your time.

Ingredients

- 2 teaspoons of vanilla extract
- 2 ½ cups of packed coconut sugar
- Sea salt
- ⅓ cup of melted coconut oil
- 3 large eggs
- 1 ½ cups of creamy or chunky peanut butter
- 2 teaspoons of baking soda
- 2 ½ cups of quick-cooking oats

Directions

- Preheat the oven to 350°F.
- Then, align 2 baking sheets with parchment paper.
- Combine the peanut butter together with the sugar and coconut oil in a mixing dish.
- Mix until well combined in an electric mixer.
- Add the eggs together with the baking soda and vanilla, mix well.

- Add the oats mix to incorporate.
- Place 2 tablespoons of dough per cookie onto the prepared baking sheets.
- Shape the cookies into rounded mound and press down lightly.
- Then, let bake for 10 minutes. Allow to cool for 10 minutes.
- Transfer to a cooling rack.
- Sprinkle with flaky sea salt.
- Serve and enjoy.

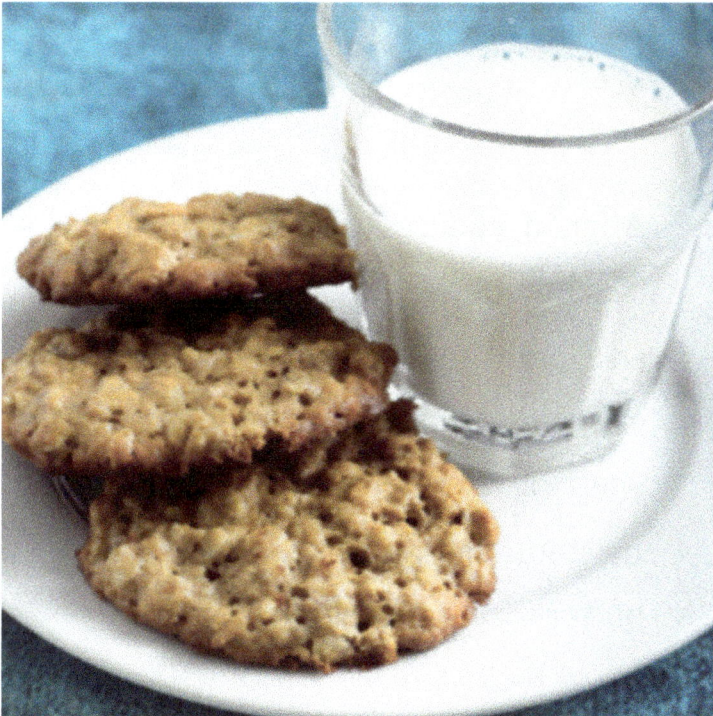

Chocolate peanut butter crispy bars

The chocolate peanut butter bars are sweetened with natural sweeteners mainly honey, baked with wholesome pantry ingredients perfect for a Mediterranean diet breakfast.

Ingredients

- ½ cup of honey
- 1 ¼ cups of whole pecans
- ½ teaspoon of flaky sea salt
- ¾ cup of creamy peanut butter
- 1 ½ cups of chocolate chips
- 3 cups of brown rice crisps

Directions

- Align a square baking dish with a strip of parchment paper
- In a large mixing bowl, combine the brown rice crisps together with 1 cup of chopped pecans. keep for later.
- In another saucepan, combine the peanut butter together with the honey.

- Warm the mixture over medium-low heat, stirring often, until steaming in 5 minutes.
- Pour the warm mixture into the bowl of rice crisps.
- Stir until the mixture is completely combined.
- Then, transfer to the lined baking dish.
- Melt the chocolate chips for 30 seconds, stirring after each one.
- Pour it over the peanut butter-crispy mixture. Spread with spatula evenly.
- Sprinkle the remaining pecans on top, then with salt.
- Refrigerate for at least 2 hours or more.
- Slice, serve and enjoy.

Healthier ginger bread cookies

Mediterranean Sea diet is a healthy choice of diet. As a result, these ginger bread cookies have all the healthy properties for a perfect Mediterranean Sea diet.

Ingredients

- ¼ teaspoon of lemon zest
- 2 teaspoons of ground cinnamon
- ¾ teaspoon of kosher salt
- ½ teaspoon of finely ground black pepper
- 2 ¼ teaspoons of lemon juice
- ½ teaspoon of baking soda
- ½ cup of powdered sugar
- ¼ teaspoon of baking powder
- ½ cup melted coconut oil
- 3 cups of whole wheat pastry flour
- ½ cup of unsulphured molasses
- ½ cup of packed coconut sugar
- 1 large egg
- Powdered sugar
- ½ teaspoon of ground cloves
- 2 teaspoons of ground ginger

Directions

- Combine the flour together with the ginger, salt, cloves, cinnamon, pepper, baking soda, and baking powder. Whisk to blended.
- Then, combine the coconut oil with molasses, whisk to combined.
- Add the coconut sugar, whisk.
- Add the egg and whisk until the mixture is thoroughly blended.
- Pour the liquid mixture into the dry, mix until combined.
- Divide the dough in half. Shape each half into a round disc about, wrap in plastic wrap.
- Refrigerate overnight.
- Preheat your oven to 350°F.
- Align 2 baking sheets with parchment paper.
- Roll out one of the discs out until ¼ thick.
- Place each cookie on a parchment-lined baking sheet.
- Bake for 11 minutes, let cool.

- Combine the powdered sugar with lemon zest and the lemon juice. Whisk to blend. Squeeze icing onto the cookies, let harden.
- Serve and enjoy.

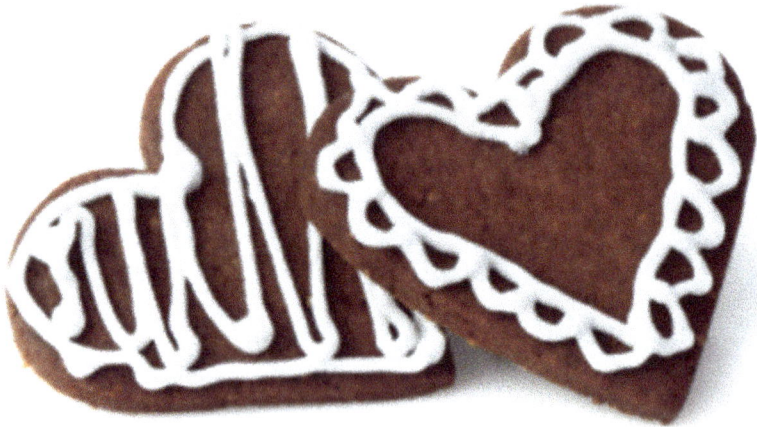

Peanut butter, banana, honey, and oat chocolate chip cookies

The ingredients of this Mediterranean diet recipe yield the highest health benefits especially the banana and oats. It is a whole meal yet perfect foe breakfast and a snack.

Ingredients

- ½ teaspoon of baking powder
- ½ cup of natural unsalted peanut butter
- 4 tablespoons of unsalted butter, melted
- 1 large egg
- ½ teaspoon of baking soda
- ½ teaspoon of ground cinnamon
- ½ cup of honey or real maple syrup
- ⅓ cup of mashed overripe banana
- Flaky sea salt
- 1 ½ cups of old-fashioned rolled oats, ground
- 1 ½ cups of old-fashioned rolled oats
- ¾ teaspoon of fine-grain sea salt
- 1 ½ cups of semi-sweet chocolate chips
- 1 teaspoon of vanilla extract

Directions

- Preheat your oven to 325°F.
- Align 2 baking sheets with parchment paper.
- Add honey to the ½ cup of lime with peanut butter until 1 cup total liquid line.
- Pour the honey and peanut butter mixture into a mixing bowl.
- Add the mashed banana together with the melted butter, whisk until to blend.
- Beat in the egg, then whisk in the vanilla together with the baking soda, baking powder, salt, and cinnamon.
- Stir in the ground oats with rolled oats, chocolate chips, and sprinkles until they are evenly combined.
- Drop the dough by the heaping tablespoon onto prepared baking sheets.
- Let bake while reversing the pans midway through until barely set within 16 minutes.
- Remove, let them cool completely on the pans.
- Serve and enjoy sprinkled with flaky salt.

Crispy baked tostones

The tostones uses green plantains as the main Mediterranean recipe ingredients with a delicious savory and salt to elevate its taste.

Ingredients

- Flaky sea salt
- 3 large unripe plantains
- 4 tablespoons avocado oil

Directions

- Start by preheating your oven to 425°F.
- Line a large baking sheet with parchment paper.
- Toss the sliced plantains with 2 tablespoons of the oil in the baking sheet.
- Disperse evenly across the pan.
- Let bake for 15 minutes, then place the pan on a heat-safe surface.
- Brush the tops of each round with oil, flip them and brush the other sides
- Sprinkle with the salt.

- Return the pan to the oven, let bake for 17 minutes, until golden.
- Season with additional salt, to taste.
- Serve and enjoy with dipping sauce.

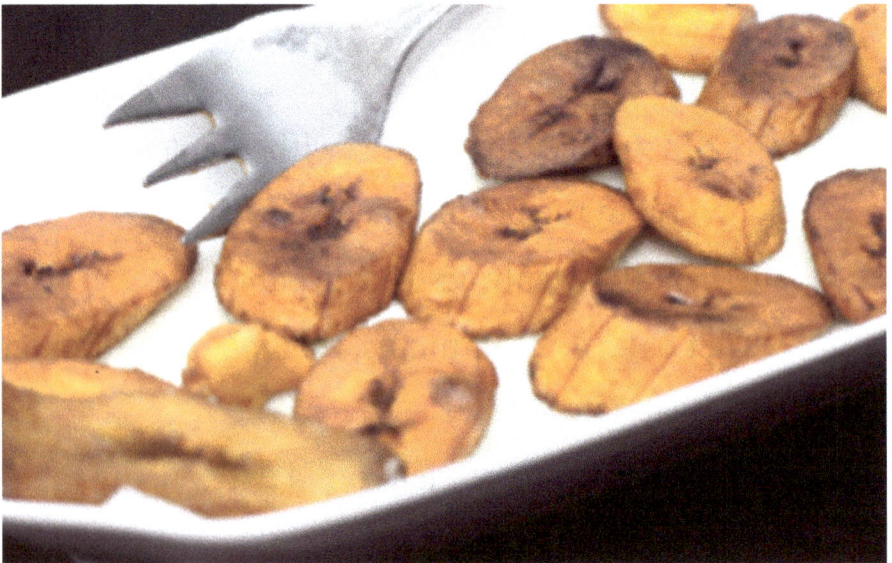

Pecan sweet potato casserole

Ingredients

- ½ stick of unsalted butter, melted
- ¼ cup of packed coconut sugar
- Pinch of fine salt
- ½ cup of milk of choice
- ¾ cup of pecan halves
- ¼ cup of maple syrup
- ½ teaspoon of vanilla extract
- 3 pounds of sweet potatoes
- 2 teaspoons of finely snipped fresh rosemary leaves
- ½ teaspoon of ground cinnamon
- ¼ teaspoon of ground nutmeg
- ½ teaspoon of fine salt
- 3 tablespoons of unsalted butter

Directions

- Preheat the oven to 425°F.
- Line a baking sheet with parchment paper.
- Grease a square baker with butter.
- Prick sweet potatoes with a fork about 5 times.

- Place the whole sweet potatoes on the prepared baking sheet, let bake for 45 minutes to 1 hour.
- Lower the heat to 350°F. Scoop the insides of potatoes into a large mixing bowl.
- Add the melted butter together with the maple syrup, vanilla, milk, nutmeg, and salt to the bowl.
- Mix until smooth and creamy.
- Scoop the mixture into the prepared baker and spread in an even layer.
- In a medium bowl, combine the softened butter together with the, sugar, pecans, rosemary, cinnamon, and salt.
- Stir until the mixture is evenly incorporated.
- Let bake for 30 minutes, until the pecans are golden and fragrant.
- Serve and enjoy.

Vegetarian succotash

This is a lovely gift for the Mediterranean Sea diet vegetarian lovers. Packed with variety of vegetables typically pecans, basil, onions, and garlic among others for a greater flavor.

Ingredients

- Pinch of cayenne
- 2 tablespoons of extra virgin olive oil
- 1 teaspoon of fine salt, divided
- Flaky sea salt
- 1 small red onion, chopped
- ¼ cup of chopped fresh basil, divided
- 1 poblano pepper, chopped
- 2 tablespoons of chopped green onion
- 1 red bell pepper, chopped
- 2 cloves garlic, pressed
- 2 cups of fresh beans
- 4 ears of fresh corn, shucked
- 2 tablespoons of butter
- Freshly ground black pepper

Directions

- Warm olive oil over medium-high heat, until starting to shimmer.
- Add the corn with ½ teaspoon of the salt.
- Let cook for 7 minutes, stirring frequently, until the corn is turning golden.
- Lower the heat, then add the onion together with the poblano, bell pepper, jalapeño, and the remaining salt.
- Stir to combine, cook, stirring often, until the onion is tender and turning translucent.
- Add the garlic, stir to combine, let cook until fragrant.
- Then, add the lima beans let cook for 2 minutes.
- Add the butter to the skillet and stir until it's mostly melted.
- Remove from the heat. Let cool briefly.
- Taste, and adjust the seasoning.
- Stir in about half of the basil, reserving some.
- Transfer the succotash to a serving plate.
- Serve and enjoy.

Mexican street corn

This corn is no ordinary corn, it is accompanied with chili powder, lime and mayonnaise for a better taste to suit the Mediterranean Sea diet taste. It works as a snack or an appetizer.

Ingredients

- ¼ teaspoon of kosher salt
- 2 ounces of finely grated Cotjia cheese
- ¼ cup of mayonnaise
- 2 tablespoons of finely chopped cilantro
- 1 ½ teaspoons of lime juice
- ½ teaspoon of chili powder
- Pinch of cayenne pepper
- 4 ears of grilled corn on the cob

Directions

- In a small bowl, combine the mayonnaise together with the lime juice, chili powder, cayenne, and salt. Stir to combined.
- In another separate bowl, mix together the cheese with the cilantro. Set both aside for later.

- Brush the mayonnaise mixture all over one ear of corn.
- Sprinkle the Cotjia mixture liberally all over, turning the corn as needed.
- Place the finished cob on a separate serving plate.
- Repeat this step for the remaining corn.
- Sprinkle a pinch of additional chili powder lightly over the corn.
- Serve and enjoy when still warm.

Best guacamole

Ingredients

- 3 tablespoons of lime juice
- ¼ cup of finely chopped fresh cilantro
- 1 teaspoon of kosher salt
- 1 small jalapeño, seeds and ribs removed
- ½ cup of finely chopped white onion
- 4 medium ripe avocados
- ¼ teaspoon of ground coriander

Directions

- Scoop the flesh of the avocados into a serving bowl.
- Then, mash up the avocado until smooth to your expectation.
- Next, add the onion together with the cilantro, coriander, jalapeño, lime juice, and salt. Stir until combine.
- Taste, and adjust the seasoning to your taste.
- Serve and enjoy.

Avocado pesto toast

Avocado is one of the few Mediterranean fruits blessed with the gift of nourishing the skin. As a result, this recipe featuring tomatoes and garlic for a flavor is adequate for your skin nourishment needs.

Ingredients

- Cooked eggs
- 2 large ripe avocados
- Freshly ground black pepper, red pepper flakes
- 2 medium cloves garlic
- 2 tablespoons of lemon juice
- Halved cherry tomatoes
- ¼ teaspoon of salt
- ¼ cup of pepitas
- ⅔ cup of packed fresh basil leaves
- 4 slices of organic bread

Directions

- Place the pepitas into a small skillet.
- Let cook over medium heat, stirring frequently until making little popping noises.

- Then, transfer to a bowl, let cool.
- Scoop avocado flesh into a bowl of a food processor.
- Place the garlic together with the lemon juice, and salt.
- Blend until smooth.
- Add the toasted pepitas with the basil leaves and pulse until the pepitas and basil are broken down.
- Taste, and adjust seasoning accordingly.
- Spread a generous amount of avocado pesto over each slice of toasted bread.
- Serve and enjoy.

Sweet potatoes and black bean tostadas

This is a complete vegetarian Mediterranean recipe with roasted sweet potatoes serve beautifully on a bed of crisp salad.

Ingredients

- Salt
- Small handful of fresh cilantro leaves, chopped
- Extra virgin olive oil
- 1 teaspoon of ground cumin
- 2 cans of black beans, rinsed and drained
- Hot sauce or salsa
- ½ cup of water
- 2 cloves garlic, pressed
- 2 ripe avocados, pitted and thinly sliced
- ½ teaspoon sea salt grinder
- 8 corn of tortillas
- 18 ounces of romaine lettuce, roughly chopped
- 1 ¾ pounds of sweet potatoes
- ⅔ cup of feta cheese crumbles
- ½ teaspoon chili powder
- ¾ cup of finely chopped red onion, divided

- 2 tablespoons of fresh lime juice

Directions

- Preheat the oven to 400°F.

- Line baking sheets with parchment paper.

- Place the sweet potatoes on baking sheets, drizzle with olive oil, and sprinkle with the chili powder and dash of salt. Toss to coat.

- Let bake for 35 minutes, or until the sweet potatoes are tender and caramelized.

- Warm olive oil over medium heat, until shimmering.

- Then, add the garlic and cumin, let cook briefly, while stirring constantly.

- Add drained beans, water and salt. Let simmer and cook for 10 minutes, stirring often.

- Remove from the heat and mash the beans, cover and set aside.

- On a baking sheet, brush both sides of each tortilla with oil.

- Arrange 4 tortillas in a single layer across each pan.

- Let bake for 12 minutes, turning until each tortilla is golden. Keep aside for later.
- In a medium serving dish, combine the chopped lettuce together with the feta, red onion, olive oil, and lime juice. Toss to combine.
- Divide the salad between 4 bowls.
- Serve and enjoy immediately.

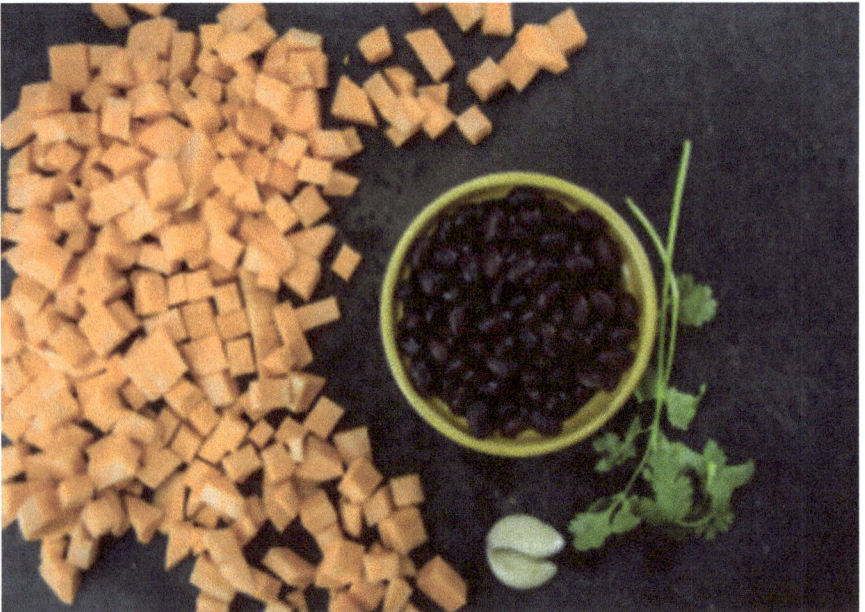

Kale, black bean, and avocado burrito bowl

Ingredients

- 3 cloves garlic, pressed
- ¼ teaspoon of salt
- 1 bunch of curly kale
- ¼ teaspoon of chili powder
- 2 tablespoons of olive oil
- ½ jalapeño, seeded and finely chopped
- ½ teaspoon of cumin
- Cherry tomatoes, sliced into thin rounds
- ¼ teaspoon of salt
- ¼ cup of lime juice
- 1 cup of brown rice, rinsed
- 1 avocado
- ½ cup of mild salsa Verde
- ¼ teaspoon of cayenne pepper
- ½ cup of fresh cilantro leaves
- Hot sauce
- 2 tablespoons of lime juice
- 2 cans of black beans, rinsed and drained

- 1 shallot, finely chopped

Directions

- Bring a big pot of water to a boil, lace in the brown rice and boil, uncovered, for 30 minutes.
- Drain any excess water, return to the pot. Let steam in the pot for 10 minutes, season with ¼ teaspoon salt and adjust accordingly.
- Whisk the lime juice together with the olive oil, chopped jalapeño, cumin, and salt.
- Toss the chopped kale with the lime marinade in a mixing bowl.
- Combine the avocado chunks, salsa Verde, cilantro, and lime juice in a food processer, blend well.
- Warm 1 tablespoon olive oil over medium-low heat.
- Sauté the shallot together with the garlic until fragrant.
- Add the beans with chili powder and cayenne pepper.

- Let cook until the beans are warmed through in 7 minutes.
- Serve and enjoy.

Sweet corn and black bean tacos

Beans are rich in protein; therefore, combining with variety of vegetables and fruits makes this recipe a perfect choice for Mediterranean Sea diet.

Ingredients

- 1 large avocado, sliced into thin strips
- Salt and black pepper
- 3 medium red radishes, thinly sliced into small strips
- ¼ cup of chopped cilantro
- 1 medium jalapeño pepper, seeded and minced
- 1 tablespoon of olive oil
- Pickled jalapeños, salsa Verde
- ¼ teaspoon of sea salt
- 2 ears of corn, shucked
- ⅔ cup of crumbled feta, to taste
- 1 medium lime, zested and juiced
- 2 cans of black beans, rinsed and drained
- 10 small round corn tortillas
- 1 tablespoon of olive oil
- 1 small yellow or white onion, chopped

- 1 tablespoon of ground cumin
- ⅓ cup of water

Directions

- Place the kernels in a medium-sized mixing bowl with jalapeño, olive oil, chopped cilantro, radishes, lime zest and juice, and sea salt. Mix well.
- Then, stir in crumbled feta, taste, and adjust.
- Warm the olive oil over medium heat.
- Add the onions with a sprinkle of salt, let cook 8 minutes, stirring occasionally.
- Add the cumin, let cook briefly while stirring.
- Pour in the beans and ⅓ cup water. Stir.
- Lower the heat, let simmer, for 5 minutes, covered.
- Smash half of the beans.
- Remove from heat, then, season with salt and pepper.
- Heat a cast iron over medium heat and warm each tortilla individually, flipping occasionally.
- Serve and enjoy.

Lemony broccoli, chickpea, and avocado pita sandwiches

Ingredients

- Pinch red pepper flakes
- 1 can of chickpeas, rinsed and drained
- 2 medium avocados
- 4 whole grain pita breads
- ⅓ cup of finely chopped red onion
- ⅓ cup of crumbled feta cheese
- ⅓ cup of oil-packed sun-dried tomatoes, rinsed and chopped
- ¼ cup of olive oil
- ¼ teaspoon of salt
- 2 tablespoons of lemon juice
- 1 ½ teaspoons of Dijon mustard
- 1 bunch of broccoli, florets removed and sliced thin
- 1 ½ teaspoons of honey
- 1 clove garlic, pressed or minced

Directions

- In a medium mixing bowl, combine broccoli, chickpea, sun-dried tomatoes, red onion, and feta cheese. Toss to combine.
- In a small mixing bowl, combine olive oil, lemon juice, Dijon mustard, honey, garlic, salt, and peppers. Whisk to emulsified.
- Taste, and adjust the seasoning accordingly.
- Pour the dressing over the broccoli chickpea salad, let toss to combine. Allow it to marinate.
- Scoop the avocado flesh into a bowl, mash until they are spreadable.
- Season with a pinch of salt.
- Warm pita bread in microwave and spread each slice with mashed avocado.
- Serve and enjoy.

Portobello mushroom and poblano pepper fajitas

Ingredients

- 2 tablespoons of fresh parsley
- ¼ cup of olive oil
- ½ lime, juiced
- 1 small jalapeño, finely chopped
- ½ teaspoon of ground cumin
- ¼ cup of lime juice
- Sea salt and black pepper
- 2 tablespoons of water
- ½ teaspoon of ground coriander
- 10 corn tortillas
- ¼ teaspoon of ground chili powder
- ⅓ cup of fresh cilantro
- 2 avocados
- Sea salt and black pepper
- 3 large Portobello mushrooms, rinsed and pat dry
- 1 medium purple onion
- 4 medium poblano peppers

- ⅔ cup of crumbled feta cheese

Directions

- Begin by tossing the slices of Portobello mushroom, poblano pepper, and onion into a large bowl.
- In a small bowl, whisk together olive oil, lime juice, jalapeno, cumin, coriander, chili powder, salt, and pepper to emulsify.
- Pour the marinade over the bowl of prepared veggies. Toss well.
- Let the veggies soak the marinate for 30 minutes.
- In a food processor, combine the avocados together with the cilantro, parsley, lime juice, and water. Blend, and season with sea salt and black pepper.
- Transfer to a small serving bowl.
- Heat a tablespoon of olive oil over medium heat.
- Add in the marinated vegetables once the olive oil is shimmering, let cook, stirring occasionally, until the peppers are tender.

- Remove from heat.
- Warm the tortillas individually in a lightly oiled pan over medium-low heat, flipping halfway through cooking.
- Stack the warmed tortillas on a plate and keep them warm under a tea towel.
- Serve and enjoy with tortillas and or avocado sauce.

Veggie breakfast sandwich

The vegetable breakfast sandwich recipe has versatile choice of toppings. It uses variety of vegetables and fruits mainly avocado.

Ingredients

- 2 teaspoons of mayonnaise
- Thinly sliced red onion
- ½ ripe avocado, mashed
- Salt and freshly ground black pepper
- 1 slice of ripe red tomato
- 1 large egg
- Small handful of arugula
- ½ teaspoon of water
- 1 teaspoon of butter or olive oil
- 2 small slices of cheddar
- 1 whole wheat muffin, sliced in half and toasted
- Several dashes of hot sauce

Directions

- Start by spreading the mayonnaise over the lower half of the toasted muffin.

- Then, spread the mashed avocado over the other half, and sprinkle it with a bit of salt and pepper.
- Heat a medium non-stick skillet over medium-high heat.
- In a bowl, scramble the egg with water and bit of salt and pepper.
- Add a pat of butter and swirl the pan to coat the bottom once the pan is hot.
- Pour in the scrambled egg and immediately swirl the egg in the bottom of the pan to make an even layer.
- Place the cheese in the center of the egg mixture, then, fold one side of the egg over the middle, then the opposite side over the middle.
- Place the cooked egg on the mayo-covered bun, topping with a slice of tomato.
- Add with several slices of red onion, a few dashes of hot sauce, and a little handful of arugula.
- Top with the remaining bun, avocado side down.

- Serve and enjoy.

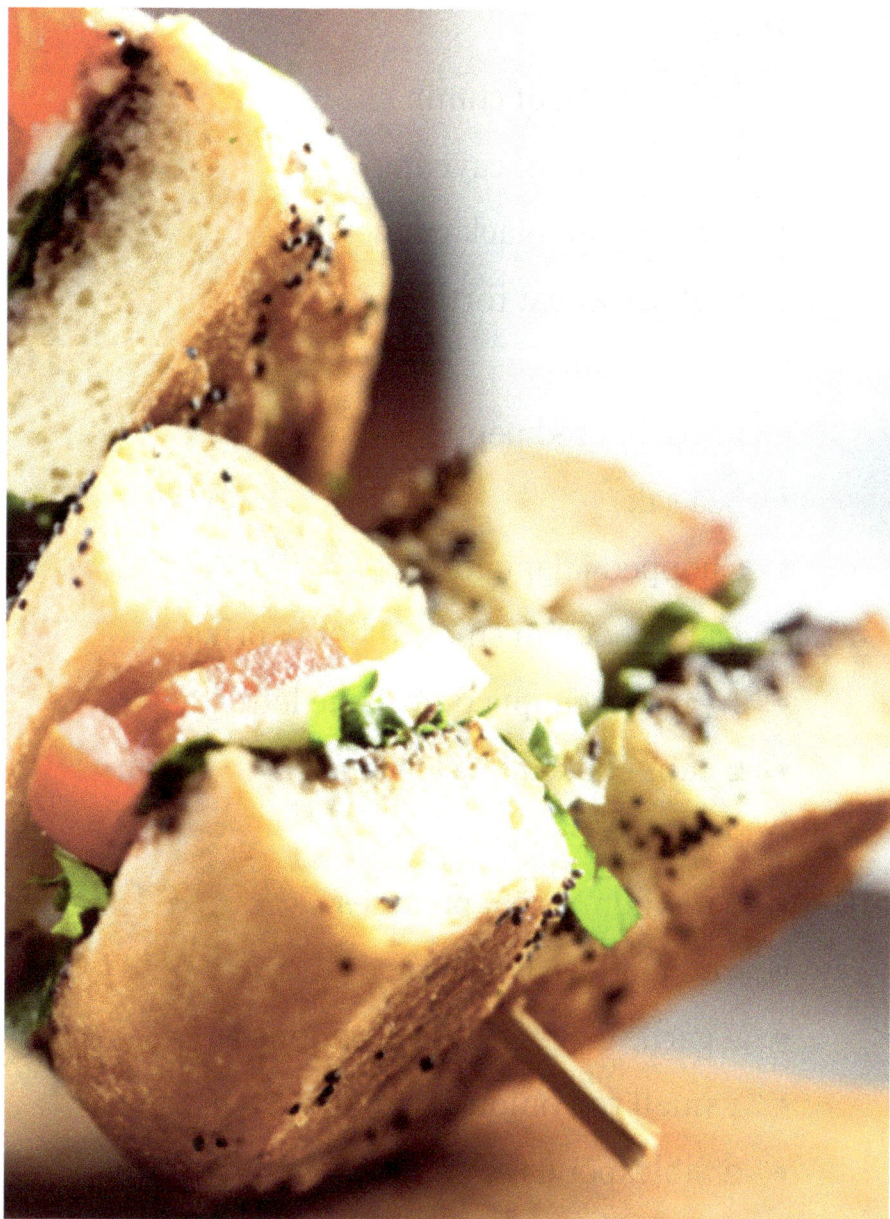

Sweet potato burrito smothered in avocado salsa Verde

Ingredients

- ½ teaspoon of cumin
- ¼ teaspoon of cayenne
- Sea salt and black pepper
- 6 whole wheat tortillas
- Sour cream
- 2 roasted red peppers
- Sea salt
- Chopped jalapeño
- ½ teaspoon of smoked hot paprika
- 1 ½ cups chopped romaine lettuce
- 2 cups cooked black beans
- 2 ripe avocados
- 2 medium sweet potatoes
- 1 cup mild salsa Verde
- 2 garlic cloves, roughly chopped
- 1 small red onion
- 2 tablespoons of extra-virgin olive oil
- 2 teaspoons of fresh jalapeño

- 1 lime, juiced
- ¼ cup of packed cilantro leaves

Directions

- Start by preheating the oven to 450°F.
- Toss the sweet potatoes together with the olive oil, smoked hot paprika, cumin, cayenne pepper, and salt and pepper.
- Place the sweet potatoes onto a large baking sheet lined with parchment paper.
- Let bake for about 45 minutes, flipping the sweet potato chunks halfway, until golden and caramelized.
- Combine the avocado flesh together with the salsa Verde, garlic, jalapeño, and lime juice in a blender. Blend.
- Add the cilantro and blend again.
- Taste, and adjust the seasoning accordingly.
- Place the tortillas on a baking sheet lined with parchment paper.
- In the middle of each tortilla, put down a couple strips of roasted red pepper, pour ⅓ cup

black beans down the center, topping with ⅓ cup of roasted sweet potato chunks.

- Let bake for 5 minutes on the middle rack, until the cheese is melted.
- Transfer each burrito to a plate, then smother in avocado sauce and sprinkle with ample romaine lettuce.
- Serve and enjoy

Simple Greek avocado sandwich

Ingredients

- 6 pitted Kalamata olives, thinly sliced
- ½ of an avocado
- 1 tablespoon of basil pesto
- Balsamic reduction
- Thinly sliced red onion
- Roasted red bell pepper
- Handful of spring mix
- 2 slices of soft whole wheat bread
- Cucumber, sliced into thin rounds

Directions

- Smash the avocado smooth enough for easy spreading.
- Spread avocado on one slice of bread.
- Spread a layer of pesto on the other slice of bread.
- Top the avocado bread with a single layer of roasted red bell pepper.
- Add a layer of cucumber slices, olives, red onion, and spring mix.

- Use a spoon to sprinkle some balsamic reduction over the lettuce.
- Place the pesto slice on top, pesto side down.
- Serve and enjoy.

Autumn couscous salad

Ingredients

- 1 ½ cups of apple juice
- 8 ounces of Israeli couscous
- ¼ cup of canola oil
- 1 tablespoon olive oil
- 1 tablespoon of parsley chopped
- ½ cup of dried currants
- 1 shallot diced
- 3 tablespoons of red wine vinegar
- kosher salt and pepper
- 1 fennel bulb diced
- 2 ½ cups of butternut squash peeled, seeded and diced
- 3 tablespoons of fresh sage chopped
- ¾ cup of dried cranberries

Directions

- Start by bringing water to boil in a medium size saucepan.
- Then, add couscous and bring back to a boil.

- Lower the heat, continue to cook for 8 minutes or until al dente.
- Drain excess water in a colander. Set aside to cool for later.
- Heat olive oil over medium high heat in a large sauté pan.
- Add the shallot let cook for 1 minute, stirring often.
- Add diced fennel, continue to cook for 5 more minutes.
- Add butternut squash together with the sage, cranberries, currants, and apple juice, let cook until butternut squash has softened.
- Season with kosher salt and pepper.
- Transfer the mixture to the bowl with the couscous, reserving some.
- In another separate small mixing bowl, mix the reserved apple juice together with the canola oil, red wine vinegar, and bit of salt and pepper.
- Add to the couscous with the parsley and stir.
- Serve and enjoy.

Garlic soup with sherry

The garlic soup with sherry draws its delicious taste from the smoky paprika and dash of dry sherry. It is purely vegetable with garlic as the main flavor with herbs.

Ingredients

- 4 eggs
- 6 cloves of garlic, peeled
- 6 cups of cubed French bread
- ¼ teaspoon of sweet pimento
- 4 tablespoons of extra virgin olive oil
- Salt to taste
- ¼ cup of minced parsley
- 6 cups of chicken broth
- 3 tablespoons of dry sherry

Directions

- Begin by heating the chicken stock in a pot.
- Sauté the garlic cloves on low heat, stirring until golden.
- Sauté the bread in the remaining olive oil until browned and crusty.

- Crush and add the garlic cloves to the broth.
- Add bread together with the paprika, sherry and salt.
- Heat the broth to a boil, lower the to medium.
- Crack each egg into a small bowl.
- Pour the eggs to rest in the soup.
- Cover the pot and poach the eggs until the whites are firm.
- Serve in bowls with an egg in each and garnish with parsley.
- Serve and enjoy.

Sautéed greens with onions and tomatoes

The sautéed greens with onions and tomatoes is a Mediterranean master of vegetables and greens. It blends in variety of kingly ingredients mainly garlic, leek, cayenne pepper, and paprika.

Ingredients

- 1 ¼ cups of snipped fresh dill
- 1 teaspoon of cayenne pepper
- 1 ¼ kg of fresh mixed tender greens.
- ¼ cup of extra virgin Greek olive oil
- 2 tablespoons of tomato paste
- 2 leeks washed well and finely chopped
- 2 garlic cloves minced
- 2 teaspoons of sweet paprika powder
- 1 ¼ cups of snipped fresh wild fennel leaves or mint leaves
- 2 large onions halved and sliced
- 1 cup of plum tomatoes peeled and finely chopped
- Salt and freshly ground pepper

Directions

- Blanch and drain the greens completely.
- Heat the olive oil in a large skillet, cook the onions with leek over medium heat, stirring, for 7 minutes.
- Add the garlic together with the tomato paste, cayenne, and paprika, stir for 3 minutes or so.
- Add the wilted greens with dill, wild fennel leaves, and tomatoes.
- Let simmer over low heat, for 20 minutes uncovered.
- Taste and adjust the seasoning with salt and cayenne.
- Pour a little fresh olive oil over the greens once they are cooked.
- Serve and enjoy.

Barbunya pilaki; beans cooked with vegetables

Ingredients

- 3 tablespoons of olive oil
- 2 cups of water
- 2 cups of dried borlotti beans
- 1 lemon, cut in wedges
- 1 medium to large onion, finely chopped
- Salt and freshly ground black pepper
- 2 medium carrots, quartered and chopped in small cubes,
- 1 can of good quality canned chopped tomatoes
- Handful of flat leaf parsley, finely chopped
- 2 teaspoons of sugar

Directions

- Start by soaking the dried borlotti beans prior to the day of cooking.
- Drain the beans, rinse and transfer and boil in a pot partially covered for 35 minutes.

- Drain any excess water, rinse the cooked beans under cold water, keep aside for later.
- Heat olive oil in the pot, then stir in the onions, sauté for 3 minutes.
- Add the carrots, and sauté for 2 more minutes.
- Stir in the canned tomatoes with sugar.
- Season with salt and freshly ground black pepper. Combine.
- Add the beans to the pot and give it a good mix. Then pour in the water.
- Bring the pot to the boil.
- Lower the heat, then cover the pan partially.
- Let simmer for 35 minutes, until the beans are cooked
- Serve and enjoy at room temperature.

Braised okra recipe

Ingredients

- 500g of fresh okra
- 2 tablespoons of red wine vinegar
- ½ a cup of olive oil
- 1 onion finely chopped
- 500g of fresh pureed tomatoes
- A handful of chopped, fresh, flat leaf parsley
- Salt and pepper

Directions

- Prepare the okra.
- Sprinkle with red wine vinegar, let rest for 1 hour in a bowl.
- Drain and rinse with cold water.
- Heat olive oil in a heavy saucepan.
- Then, sauté onion over a low heat until to soften.
- Add the okra and toss in the olive oil together with the onion mixture for 5 minutes.
- Add the tomatoes with parsley, season to taste.
- Bring the mixture to a boil on high heat.

- Let simmer for 30 minutes on a low heat.
- Once the okra is tender serve and enjoy with crusty bread.

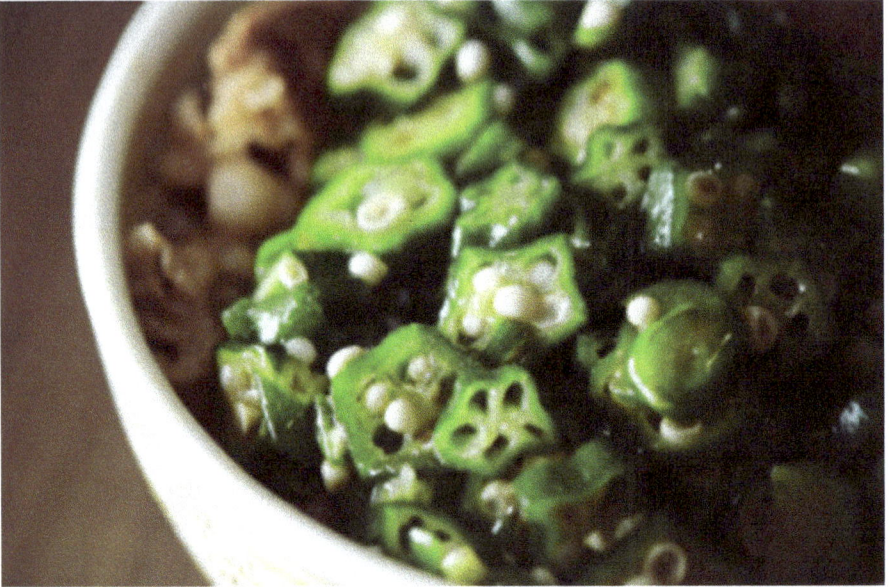

Louvi black eyed peas

Ingredients

- 1 teaspoon of flour
- 250g of black eyed beans
- 3 tablespoons of parsley, finely chopped
- 3 tablespoons of parsley, finely chopped
- 1 bunch of silver beet or chard
- 1/3 cup of lemon juice
- 1 medium onion, finely chopped
- Freshly ground black pepper
- 1 tablespoon of dill, finely chopped
- 1 spring onion, finely chopped
- 1 clove garlic, finely chopped
- ¼ cup olive oil
- 1 tablespoon of dill or fennel fronds
- Salt
- 4 cups of water

Directions

- Place black eyed beans in a pot and boil for 15 minutes.
- Drain any excess water.

- Then, sauté the onion with garlic in olive oil, then add silver beet and stir.
- Add the black eyed peas, let season with salt and pepper.
- Add water to cover all ingredients.
- Bring to boil, lower the heat, then simmer until the beans are soft.
- Toward the end add the parsley and dill and mix.
- Dissolve the flour in the lemon juice.
- Add to the mixture. Cook for a few more minutes.
- Serve and enjoy.

Greek style zucchini blossoms

Ingredients

- 2/3 cup of chopped parsley
- 1 cup olive oil
- Salt and pepper
- 1 cup of chopped onion
- 1 cup of chopped chives
- 3 tablespoons of chopped fresh mint leaves
- 3 cloves, minced garlic
- 3 cups of yogurt
- 25 zucchini blossoms
- 1 cup of grated zucchini
- 1 cup of bulgur
- 2/3 cup of raisins
- 1 teaspoon of chili pepper
- 1 ½ cups of water
- ½ cup of pine nuts

Directions

- Heat half of the olive oil over medium heat and sauté the onion, chives, and garlic for 5 minutes, or until soft.

- Add the zucchini together with the bulgur, raisins, chili pepper, and 1 cup water.
- Lower the heat, then let simmer for 10 minutes.
- Add the pine nuts, mint, and dill to the stuffing when the heat is off.
- Season with salt, stir, and adjust accordingly.
- Stuff each blossom using a spoon.
- Fold the top over and place on their sides in an earthenware casserole.
- Pour the remaining olive oil and ½ cup water.
- Cover the dish and place in the oven.
- Let bake for I hour or so.
- Serve and enjoy hot or cold, according to your liking.

Mushroom, chorizo, and haloumi tacos

This recipe has unforgettable combination of a true and healthy Mediterranean Sea diet vegetables. It is quite wonderful with homemade tortillas.

Ingredients

- 8 tortillas, medium-sized and warmed in a pan
- 500g of button mushrooms
- 1 tablespoon of chilies, finely chopped
- 3 tablespoons of olive oil
- 1 teaspoon of salt
- 125g of chorizo sausage
- 200g of haloumi cheese
- 1 teaspoon of black pepper
- 1 tablespoon of coriander, finely chopped
- 1 pinch of oregano, dried

Directions

- Combine the mushrooms together with the olive oil, salt, pepper, and oregano in a bowl.
- Place on baking tray and cook in an oven heated to 400°F for 35 minutes.
- Remove, let cool briefly.

- Preheat a little oil, cook the chorizo on a medium high heat briefly until crispy. Set aside.
- In the same pan, fry the halloumi for 2 minutes on each side until, browned.
- Cut the haloumi into small even slices.
- Combine the mushrooms, chorizo and haloumi in a separate bowl.
- Pace 3 tablespoons of the mushroom mixture into a warmed tortilla.
- Garnish with fresh chilies and coriander.
- Serve and enjoy.

Chicory and beans

Ingredients

- Olive oil
- 3 medium heads of chicory
- Salt
- 3 cloves of garlic
- 1 small can of cannellini
- 1 pepperoncino

Directions

- Boil the chicory in salted water for 10 minutes, or until fully tender.
- Drain any water, reserving some for later.
- Squeeze dry and chop the chicory roughly.
- In a large sauté pan, lightly brown the garlic in abundant olive oil, adding the pepperoncino or red pepper flakes for a few moments at the end.
- Remove both garlic and pepperoncino.
- Add the chopped chicory to the seasoned oil and let it simmer for 5 minutes.
- Then add the canned beans with a ladleful of the reserved cooking water. Mix well.

- Let the mixture simmer again briefly.

- Taste, and adjust the seasoning.

- Serve and enjoy with a drizzle of olive oil.

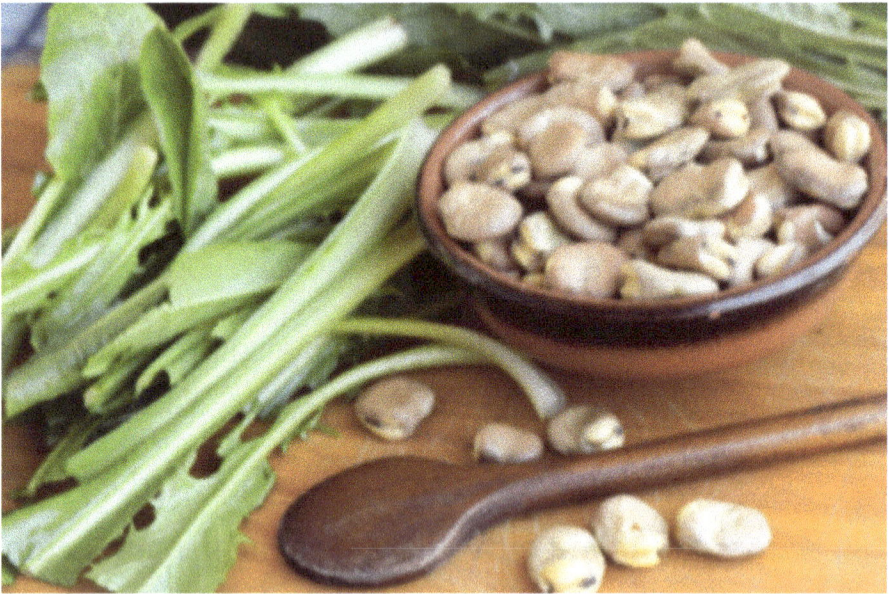

Smoked salmon with poached eggs on the toast

Ingredients

- 2 eggs, poached
- Splash of Kikkoman soy sauce
- 2 slices of bread toasted
- 1 tablespoon of thinly sliced scallions
- ½ large avocado smashed
- ¼ teaspoon of freshly squeezed lemon juice
- Pinch of kosher salt and cracked black pepper
- Microgreens
- 3.5 oz. of smoked salmon

Directions

- Smash the avocado in a small mixing bowl.
- Add the lemon juice and a pinch of salt, mix well and keep.
- Poach the eggs, when they are sitting in the ice bath, toast the bread.
- Spread the avocado on both slices of toasted bread, then add the smoked salmon to each slice.

- Transfer the poached eggs to their respective toasts.
- Hit with a splash of Kikkoman soy sauce and some cracked pepper.
- Place slice of tomato on each toast.
- Serve and enjoy.

Vegetarian potato skin egg boats

Ingredients

- 1 cup of shredded cheddar cheese
- 4 russet potatoes
- Fresh or dried chives
- 2 tablespoons of olive oil
- 8 large eggs
- Coarse kosher salt and freshly ground black pepper
- 2 teaspoons of smoked paprika

Directions

- Begin by preheating your oven ready to 450°F.
- Place potatoes on a baking sheet and pierce each one a few times with a fork.
- Let bake for 60 minutes.
- Remove, and let cool enough to handle.
- Raise the heat to 475°F.
- Slice each potato in half lengthwise.
- Scoop out the flesh, leaving ¼ inch of potato around the edge.

- Brush both sides lightly with olive oil and bake cut side down for 16 minutes, flipping halfway through.
- Lower the heat to 375°F.
- Season the inside of the potato skins with salt, pepper, and smoked paprika.
- Divide cheese evenly amongst the potatoes, then crack one egg into each.
- Sprinkle with chopped chives.
- Return the potatoes to the oven, let bake until the yolks jiggle slightly in 17 minutes or so.
- Serve and enjoy.

Baked eggs skillet with avocado and spicy tomatoes

Ingredients

- Vege-Sal and fresh-ground black pepper
- 1 10 oz. can of tomatoes
- 1 ripe avocado, sliced lengthwise
- 4 eggs

Directions

- Preheat your oven to 400F.
- Break eggs into individual ramekins and let the eggs come to room temperature.
- Brush a medium sized ovenproof pan with oil.
- Add the tomatoes, start to simmer over medium heat.
- Turn off the heat once all the liquid has evaporated from the tomatoes
- Arrange the avocado slices like spokes of a wheel in the pan.
- Place each egg between two avocado slices, spacing them evenly.

- Season with salt and fresh-ground black pepper.
- Place the skillet into the pre-heated oven, let bake until whites are completely set and the yolks are done in 10 - 13 minutes.
- Serve and enjoy hot.

Chard, mozzarella, and feta egg bake

Ingredients

- 8 eggs, beaten
- ¼ cup of sliced green onions
- 8 oz. of Swiss chard leaves, sliced into thick ribbons
- 1 teaspoon of Spike Seasoning
- 2 teaspoon of olive oil
- 3/4 cup of Mozzarella cheese
- Salt and fresh ground black pepper
- ½ cup of crumbled Feta cheese

Directions

- Preheat your oven to 375°F.
- Spray a glass casserole dish with olive oil.
- Cut stems off the chard leaves and discard stems.
- Stack up the leaves in a pile and cut the chard into ribbons.
- Then, heat olive oil in a heavy non-stick frying pan.

- Add the chard ribbons all at once, let cook while stirring until the chard has wilted and slightly softened in 3 minutes.
- Layer the wilted chard together with Mozzarella cheese, and Feta cheese in the bottom of the casserole dish sprinkled with green onions.
- Beat the eggs with the spike seasoning, salt, and pepper.
- Pour over the chard.
- Let bake until the egg bake is set and starting to lightly brown within 40 minutes.
- Serve and enjoy with a dollop of sour cream.

Bacon spinach and sweet potato frittata

Ingredients

- 1 cup of shredded cheddar cheese
- ¼ lb. of bacon
- large handful of baby spinach
- ½ cup of milk
- 1 large sweet potato peeled and cut into disks
- Kosher salt to taste
- 1 med onion diced
- 6 eggs

Directions

- Cook the bacon in a large oven-proof skillet over high heat.
- When ready, remove the bacon to a paper towel lined plate, keep aside.
- Lower the heat to medium, then add the onions to the same skillet with the bacon drippings.
- Let the onions cook for 2 minutes, then add the potato slices.
- Sprinkle with salt, let cook for 3 minutes on each side.

- Whisk the eggs together with the milk.
- Add salt and pepper, set aside for later.
- Preheat your oven to broiler low.
- When the potatoes are slightly browned and soft, sprinkle them with baby spinach.
- Pour the egg mixture on top and then sprinkle with the cooked bacon.
- Top with shredded cheese, let continue to cook over medium low heat, until the eggs start to set in 10 minutes.
- After 8 minutes, lift the edges of the eggs to allow the liquid to run down underneath.
- Transfer the pan to the oven.
- Broil until lightly browned.
- Slice, serve and enjoy.

www.ingramcontent.com/pod-product-compliance
Lightning Source LLC
Chambersburg PA
CBHW050747030426
42336CB00012B/1696